Table of Contents

Introduction 3
Liver 3
    Structure Of The Liver 4
    Purpose Of The Liver 4
    Liver Regeneration 6
    Diseases That Can Develop In The Liver 7
    Symptoms Of Liver Conditions 9
    How To Keep Your Liver Healthy 11
    Liver Function Tests 11
    Common Liver Function Tests 13
    Need For Liver Function Test 15
    How To Prepare For A Liver Function Test 16
    How A Liver Function Test Is Performed 17
    Risks Of A Liver Function Test 17
    Symptoms Of Fatty Liver 19
    Causes 20
    Diagnosing Of Fatty Liver 21
Liver Biopsy 23
    Treatment For Fatty Liver 23
    Home Remedies 24
Diet For Fatty Liver Disease 25

- Types Of Fatty Liver Disease 26
- Risk Factors 28
- Stages Of Fatty Liver 29
- Prevention 30

Liver Cancer 31
- Different Types Of Primary Liver Cancer 32
- Symptoms Of Liver Cancer 33
- People At Risk Of Liver Cancer 34
- Liver Cancer Diagnosis 35
- Liver Cancer Treatment 37
- Liver Cancer Prevention 40
- Reduce Your Risk Of Cirrhosis 41

Liver Detox Diet 42
- Foods To Help Fatty Liver Reversal 52
- Foods And Drinks That You Should Eat For A Fatty Liver 53
- Foods To Avoid If You Have A Fatty Liver 55

Recipes 57
- Conclusion 62

Introduction

The liver is your body's largest internal organ.It's responsible for more than 500 different functions in the body. One of these functions is detoxification and neutralizing toxins.Knowing that the liver is a detoxification organ, you might think doing a liver cleanse could help your body recover faster after a big weekend, give your body that much-needed health kick, or boost your metabolism so you can lose weight faster. That's what all those "liver cleanses" on the market claim they can do. But truth be told, you're likely wasting your money and could be doing your body more harm than good. The reality is that toxins are everywhere in our environment, and our bodies have the built-in capacity to defend against these toxins naturally. Of course, there are things you can do to improve your health and support healthy liver function.

Liver

Your liver is your body's largest solid organ. On average, it weighs around 3 pounds in adulthood and is roughly the size of a football. This organ is vital to the body's metabolic functions and immune system. Without a functioning liver, a person cannot survive. The liver's position is mostly in the right upper portion of the stomach, a portion of the liver goes into the left upper abdomen as well.

Structure Of The Liver

The liver is a half-moon shaped organ that's fairly straight on the bottom. It's tilted slightly in the body's cavity, with the left portion above the stomach and the right portion above the first part of the small intestine. The liver has two main portions, or lobes. Each lobe is further divided into eight segments. Each segment has an estimated 1,000 lobules, or small lobes. Each of these lobules has a small tube (duct) that flows toward the common hepatic duct. Compared to the rest of the body, the liver has a significant amount of blood flowing through it an estimated 13 percent of the body's blood is in the liver at any given time.

Purpose Of The Liver

The liver's major functions are in the metabolic processes of the body. These include:

- Breaking down or converting substances
- Extracting energy
- Making toxins less harmful to the body and removing them from the bloodstream

The liver does this by receiving blood with nutrients from the digestive organs via a vein known as the portal vein. The many cells of the liver, known as hepatocytes, accept and filter this blood. They act as little sorting centers, determining:

- Which nutrients should be processed?
- What should be stored
- What should be eliminated via the stool
- What should go back to the blood

The liver stores vitamins as well as minerals such as copper and iron, releasing them if the body needs them. The liver also helps to break down fats in a person's diet. It either stores fats or releases them as energy. It also manufactures an estimated 800 to 1,000 milliliters of bile a day. This bile is transported via a bile duct to the small intestine. The small intestine uses the bile to further break down fats. Any extra bile is stored in the gallbladder. The liver breaks down proteins as well. The by-product of this process is called ammonia, which can be toxic to the body in large amounts. The liver turns the toxic ammonia into a substance called urea. The liver releases this into the blood where the kidneys excrete it via the urine. The liver also breaks down alcohol in the blood as well as many medications you take. As if these functions weren't enough, the liver also plays major roles in the following:

- Creating immune system factors that can fight against infection
- Creating proteins responsible for blood clotting
- Breaking down old and damaged red blood cells
- Storing extra blood sugar as glycogen

When taking these factors into consideration, its easy to see how important the liver is to a person's health.

Liver Regeneration

The liver is truly an amazing organ in that it has the capacity to regenerate. This means that after an injury or surgery to remove tissue, the liver tissue can grow back to a certain extent. The liver starts growing back by having the existing cells enlarge. Then, new liver cells start to multiply.Within a week after removing two-thirds of the liver, the liver can return to the same weight it was before surgery. The liver has been known to regenerate completely after as many as 12 partial liver removal surgeries.

Diseases That Can Develop In The Liver

There are many types of diseases that can affect the liver and its functions. Some have successful treatments while others do not. Examples of common conditions that affect the liver include:

Autoimmune Hepatitis

This condition causes the body's immune system to attack itself and destroy healthy liver tissue. Autoimmune hepatitis can lead to cirrhosis and other liver damage.

Biliary Atresia

Biliary atresia is a condition that adversely affects a person's bile ducts and bile flow when they're an infant. If left untreated, the condition can cause liver scarring and affect liver tissue. Fortunately, there are treatments available for the condition.

Cirrhosis

Cirrhosis is a condition where scar tissue replaces healthy liver tissue. A number of conditions can cause cirrhosis. These include long-term excessive alcohol use, chronic hepatitis, or rare genetic disorders, such as Wilson's disease.

Hemochromatosis

This condition causes an excess of iron to build up in the body. Too much iron can damage the liver.

Hepatitis A

Viral hepatitis refers to a viral infection that causes liver inflammation. The hepatitis types have different letters, including A, B, C, D, and E. Each has different causes and severity. Hepatitis A is more common in developing countries that lack clean drinking water and have poor sanitation systems. Most people can recover from hepatitis A without liver failure or long-term complications.

Hepatitis B

Hepatitis B can cause a short- or long-term infection. In U.S. adults, the disease is most commonly spread through sexual contact. However, a person can also get it through sharing needles or accidentally injecting themselves with a contaminated needle. The condition can cause serious complications, including liver failure and cancer. There's a vaccination against the disease to prevent it.

Hepatitis C

Hepatitis C can be an acute or chronic infection. It's most commonly spread by coming in contact with blood containing the hepatitis C virus, such as through sharing unclean needles to inject drugs or apply tattoos. Less commonly, unprotected sexual contact with an infected person can transmit the infection, too.This condition can cause inflammation that can lead to cirrhosis, liver failure, and liver cancer.

Nonalcoholic Fatty Liver Disease And NASH

These are conditions where fat builds up in the liver. An excess of fat can damage the liver, causing inflammation. Nonalcoholic steatohepatitis (NASH) is a form of nonalcoholic fatty liver disease that causes scarring or fibrosis. People who are obese and have conditions related to obesity, such as type 2 diabetes, are more likely to have this disease.

Symptoms Of Liver Conditions

There are more than 100 types of liver diseases. Many conditions begin as flu-like symptoms and progress to more severe signs of liver damage, such as jaundice and dark-colored urine. Other symptoms of liver problems include:

- Fatigue
- Loss of appetite

- Nausea
- Vomiting
- Joint pain
- Stomach discomfort or pain
- Nose bleeds
- Abnormal blood vessels on the skin (spider angiomas)
- Itchy skin
- Weakness
- A low sex drive

More serious symptoms include:

- Yellowing of the skin and eyes (jaundice)
- Confusion and difficulty thinking clearly
- Abdominal swelling (ascites)
- Swelling of the legs (edema)
- Impotence
- Gynecomastia (when males start to develop breast tissue)
- Enlarged liver (hepatomegaly)
- Dark urine
- Pale-colored stools

If you're experiencing any of the symptoms mentioned above, see your doctor immediately.

How To Keep Your Liver Healthy

These lifestyle changes can help you keep your liver healthy:

- Get vaccinated for hepatitis a and hepatitis b
- Practice safe sex with a condom
- Don't share needles or personal care items (razors, toothbrushes, etc.)
- Exercise regularly
- Talk to your doctor about any medications you're taking as they may affect your liver
- Limit the amount of alcohol you consume since it takes a lot for your liver to breakdown the toxins from alcohol
- Maintain a healthy diet with fiber and fatty fishes

Liver Function Tests

Liver function tests, also known as liver chemistries, help determine the health of your liver by measuring the levels of proteins, liver enzymes, and bilirubin in your blood. A liver function test is often recommended in the following situations:

- To check for damage from liver infections, such as hepatitis B and hepatitis C
- To monitor the side effects of certain medications known to affect the liver

- If you already have a liver disease, to monitor the disease and how well a particular treatment is working
- If you're experiencing the symptoms of a liver disorder
- If you have certain medical conditions such as high triglycerides, diabetes, high blood pressure, or anemia
- If you drink alcohol heavily
- 08- if you have gallbladder disease

Many tests can be performed on the liver. Certain tests can reflect different aspects of liver function. Commonly used tests to check liver abnormalities are tests checking:

- Alanine transaminase (ALT)
- Aspartate aminotransferase (AST)
- Alkaline phosphatase (ALP)
- Albumin
- Bilirubin

The ALT and AST tests measure enzymes that your liver releases in response to damage or disease. The albumin test measures how well the liver creates albumin, while the bilirubin test measures how well it disposes of bilirubin.ALP can be used to evaluate the bile duct system of the liver. Having abnormal results on any of these liver tests typically requires follow up to determine the cause of the abnormalities. Even mildly elevated results can be associated with liver disease. However, these enzymes can also be found in other places besides the liver. Talk to your doctor about the results of your liver function test and what they may mean for you.

Common Liver Function Tests

Liver function tests are used to measure specific enzymes and proteins in your blood.Depending on the test, either higher or lower-than-normal levels of these enzymes or proteins can indicate a problem with your liver.Some common liver function tests include:

Alanine transaminase (ALT) test: Alanine transaminase (ALT) is used by your body to metabolize protein. If the liver is damaged or not functioning properly, ALT can be released into the blood.This causes ALT levels to increase. A higher than normal result on this test can be a sign of liver damage. According to the American College of Gastroenterology, an ALT above 25 IU/L (international units per liter) in females and 33 IU/L in male's typically requires further testing and evaluation.

Aspartate aminotransferase (AST) test: Aspartate aminotransferase (AST) is an enzyme found in several parts of your body, including the heart, liver, and muscles.Since AST levels aren't as specific for liver damage as ALT, it's usually measured together with ALT to check for liver problems. When the liver is damaged, AST can be released into the bloodstream.A high result on an AST test might indicate a problem with the liver or muscles. The normal range for AST is typically up to 40 IU/L in adults and may be higher in infants and young children.

Alkaline phosphatase (ALP) test: Alkaline phosphatase (ALP) is an enzyme found in your bones, bile ducts, and liver. An ALP test is typically ordered in combination with several other tests. High levels of ALP may indicate liver inflammation, blockage of the bile ducts, or a bone disease. Children and adolescents may have elevated levels of ALP because their bones are growing.Pregnancy can also raise ALP levels.The normal range for ALP is typically up to 120 U/L in adults.

Albumin Test: Albumin is the main protein made by your liver.It performs many important bodily functions. For example, albumin:

- Stops fluid from leaking out of your blood vessels
- Nourishes your tissues
- Transports hormones, vitamins, and other substances throughout your body

An albumin test measures how well your liver is making this particular protein. A low result on this test can indicate that your liver isn't functioning properly. The normal range for albumin is 3.5–5.0 grams per deciliter (g/dL). However, low albumin can also be a result of poor nutrition, kidney disease, infection, and inflammation.

Bilirubin test: Bilirubin is a waste product from the breakdown of red blood cells. It's ordinarily processed by the liver. It passes through the liver before being excreted through your stool. A damaged liver can't properly process bilirubin. This leads to an abnormally high level of bilirubin in the blood. A high result on the bilirubin test may indicate that the liver isn't functioning properly. The normal range for total bilirubin is typically 0.1–1.2 milligrams per deciliter (mg/dL). There are certain inherited diseases that raise bilirubin levels, but the liver function is normal.

Need For Liver Function Test

Liver tests can help determine if your liver is working correctly. The liver performs a number of vital bodily functions, such as:

- Removing contaminants from your blood
- Converting nutrients from the foods you eat

- Storing minerals and vitamins
- Regulating blood clotting
- Producing cholesterol, proteins, enzymes, and bile
- Making factors that fight infection
- Removing bacteria from your blood
- Processing substances that could harm your body
- Maintaining hormone balances
- Regulating blood sugar levels

Problems with the liver can make a person very sick and can even be life-threatening.

How To Prepare For A Liver Function Test

Your doctor will give you complete instructions on how to prepare for the blood sample portion of the test. Certain medications and foods may affect levels of these enzymes and proteins in your blood. Your doctor may ask you to avoid some types of medications, or they may ask you to avoid eating anything for a period of time before the test. Be sure to continue drinking water prior to the test. You may want to wear a shirt with sleeves that can easily be rolled up to make it easier to collect the blood sample.

How A Liver Function Test Is Performed

You may have your blood drawn in a hospital or at a specialized testing facility. To administer the test:

- The healthcare provider will clean your skin before the test to decrease the likelihood that any microorganisms on your skin will cause an infection.
- They'll likely wrap an elastic strap on your arm. This will help your veins become more visible. They'll use a needle to draw samples of blood from your arm.
- After the draw, the healthcare provider will place some gauze and a bandage over the puncture site. Then they'll send the blood sample to a laboratory for testing.

Risks Of A Liver Function Test

Blood draws are routine procedures and rarely cause any serious side effects. However, the risks of giving a blood sample can include:

- Bleeding under the skin, or hematoma
- Excessive bleeding
- Fainting
- Infection

After A Liver Function Test

After the test, you can usually leave and go about your life as usual. However, if you feel faint or lightheaded during the blood draw, you should rest before you leave the testing facility. The results of these tests may not tell your doctor exactly which condition you have or the degree of any liver damage, but they might help your doctor determine the next steps. Your doctor will call you with the results or discuss them with you at a follow-up appointment. In general, if your results indicate a problem with your liver function, your doctor will review your medications and your past medical history to help determine the cause. If you drink alcohol heavily, then you'll need to stop drinking. If your doctor identifies that a medication is causing the elevated liver enzymes, then they'll advise you to stop the medication. Your doctor may decide to test you for hepatitis, other infections, or other diseases that can affect the liver. They may also choose to do imaging, like an ultrasound or CT scan. They may recommend a liver biopsy to evaluate the liver for fibrosis, fatty liver disease, or other liver conditions.

Fatty Liver

Fatty liver is also known as hepatic steatosis. It happens when fat builds up in the liver. Having small amounts of fat in your liver is normal, but too much can become a health problem. Your liver is the second largest organ in your body. It helps process nutrients from food and drinks and filters harmful substances from your blood. Too much fat in your liver can cause liver inflammation, which can damage your liver and create scarring. In severe cases, this scarring can lead to liver failure. When fatty liver develops in someone who drinks a lot of alcohol, it's known as alcoholic fatty liver disease (AFLD). In someone who doesn't drink a lot of alcohol, it's known as non-alcoholic fatty liver disease (NAFLD). According to researchers in the World Journal of Gastroenterology, NAFLD affects up to 25 to 30 percent of people in the United States and Europe.

Symptoms Of Fatty Liver

In many cases, fatty liver causes no noticeable symptoms. But you may feel tired or experience discomfort or pain in the upper right side of your abdomen. Some people with fatty liver disease develop complications, including liver scarring. Liver scarring is known as liver fibrosis. If you develop severe liver fibrosis, it's known as cirrhosis. Cirrhosis may cause symptoms such as:

- Loss of appetite
- Weight loss

- Weakness
- Fatigue
- Nosebleeds
- Itchy skin
- Yellow skin and eyes
- Web-like clusters of blood vessels under your skin
- Abdominal pain
- Abdominal swelling
- Swelling of your legs
- Breast enlargement in men
- Confusion

Causes

Fatty liver develops when your body produces too much fat or doesn't metabolize fat efficiently enough. The excess fat is stored in liver cells, where it accumulates and causes fatty liver disease. This build-up of fat can be caused by a variety of things. For example, drinking too much alcohol can cause alcoholic fatty liver disease.This is the first stage of alcohol-related liver disease.In people who don't drink a lot of alcohol, the cause of fatty liver disease is less clear. One or more of the following factors may play a role:

- Obesity

- High blood sugar
- Insulin resistance
- High levels of fat, especially triglycerides, in your blood

Less common causes include:

- Pregnancy
- Rapid weight loss
- Some types of infections, such as hepatitis c
- Side effects from some types of medications, such as methotrexate (trexall), tamoxifen (nolvadex), amiodorone (pacerone), and valproic acid (depakote)
- Exposure to certain toxins

Certain genes may also raise your risk of developing fatty liver.

Diagnosing Of Fatty Liver

To diagnose fatty liver, your doctor will take your medical history, conduct a physical exam, and order one or more tests.

Medical history: If your doctor suspects that you might have fatty liver, they will likely ask you questions about:

- Your family medical history, including any history of liver disease
- Your alcohol consumption and other lifestyle habits

- Any medical conditions that you might have
- Any medications that you might take
- Recent changes in your health

If you've been experiencing fatigue, loss of appetite, or other unexplained symptoms, let your doctor know.

Physical exam: To check for liver inflammation, your doctor may palpate or press on your abdomen. If your liver is enlarged, they might be able to feel it.However, it's possible for your liver to be inflamed without being enlarged. Your doctor might not be able to tell if your liver is inflamed by touch.

Blood tests: In many cases, fatty liver disease is diagnosed after blood tests show elevated liver enzymes. For example, your doctor may order the alanine aminotransferase test (ALT) and aspartate aminotransferase test (AST) to check your liver enzymes. These tests might be recommended if you've developed signs or symptoms of liver disease, or they might be ordered as part of routine blood work. Elevated liver enzymes are a sign of liver inflammation.Fatty liver disease is one potential cause of liver inflammation, but it's not the only one. If you test positive for elevated liver enzymes, your doctor will likely order additional tests to identify the cause of the inflammation.

Imaging studies: Your doctor may use one or more of the following imaging tests to check for excess fat or other problems with your liver:

- Ultrasound exam
- Ct scan
- Mri scan

They might also order a test known as vibration-controlled transient elastography (VCTE, FibroScan). This test uses low-frequency sound waves to measure liver stiffness. It can help check for scarring.

Liver Biopsy

A liver biopsy is considered the best way to determine the severity of liver disease. During a liver biopsy, a doctor will insert a needle into your liver and remove a piece of tissue for examination. They will give you a local anesthetic to lessen the pain. This test can help determine if you have fatty liver disease, as well as liver scarring.

Treatment For Fatty Liver

Currently, no medications have been approved to treat fatty liver disease. More research is needed to develop and test medications to treat this condition. In many cases, lifestyle changes can help reverse fatty liver disease. For example, your doctor might advise you to:

- Limit or avoid alcohol
- Take steps to lose weight
- Make changes to your diet

If you've developed complications, your doctor might recommend additional treatments. To treat cirrhosis, for example, they might prescribe:

- Lifestyle changes
- Medications
- Surgery

Cirrhosis can lead to liver failure. If you develop liver failure, you might need a liver transplant.

Home Remedies

Lifestyle changes are the first-line treatment for fatty liver disease. Depending on your current condition and lifestyle habits, it might help to:

- Lose weight
- Reduce your alcohol intake

- Eat a nutrient-rich diet that's low in excess calories, saturated fat, and trans fats
- Get at least 30 minutes of exercise most days of the week

According to the Mayo Clinic, some evidence suggests that vitamin E supplements might help prevent or treat liver damage caused by fatty liver disease. However, more research is needed. There are some health risks associated with consuming too much vitamin E. Always talk to your doctor before you try a new supplement or natural remedy. Some supplements or natural remedies might put stress on your liver or interact with medications you're taking.

Diet For Fatty Liver Disease

If you have fatty liver disease, your doctor might encourage you to adjust your diet to help treat the condition and lower your risk of complications. For example, they might advise you to do the following:

- Eat a diet that's rich in plant-based foods, including fruits, vegetables, legumes, and whole grains.

- Limit your consumption of refined carbohydrates, such as sweets, white rice, white bread, other refined grain products.
- Limit your consumption of saturated fats, which are found in red meat and many other animal products.
- Avoid trans fats, which are present in many processed snack foods.
- Avoid alcohol.

Your Doctor May Encourage You To Cut Calories From Your Diet To Lose Weight.

Types Of Fatty Liver Disease

There Are Two Main Types Of Fatty Liver Disease: nonalcoholic and alcoholic. Nonalcoholic fatty liver disease (NAFLD) includes simple nonalcoholic fatty liver, nonalcoholic steatohepatitis (NASH), and acute fatty liver of pregnancy (AFLP). Alcoholic fatty liver disease (AFLD) includes simple AFLD and alcoholic steatohepatitis (ASH).

Nonalcoholic Fatty Liver Disease (NAFLD): Nonalcoholic fatty liver disease (NAFLD) occurs when fat builds up in the liver of people who don't drink a lot of alcohol. If you have excess fat in your liver and no history of heavy alcohol use, your doctor may diagnose you with NAFLD. If there's no inflammation or other complications along with the build-up of fat, the condition is known as simple nonalcoholic fatty liver.

Nonalcoholic Steatohepatitis (NASH): Nonalcoholic steatohepatitis (NASH) is a type of NAFLD. It occurs when a build-up of excess fat in the liver is accompanied by liver inflammation. If you have excess fat in your liver, your liver is inflamed, and you have no history of heavy alcohol use, your doctor may diagnose you with NASH. When left untreated, NASH can cause scarring of your liver. In severe cases, this can lead to cirrhosis and liver failure.

Acute Fatty Liver Of Pregnancy (AFLP): Acute fatty liver of pregnancy (AFLP) is a rare but serious complication of pregnancy. The exact cause is unknown. When AFLP develops, it usually appears in the third trimester of pregnancy. If left untreated, it poses serious health risks to the mother and growing baby. If you're diagnosed with AFLP, your doctor will want to deliver your baby as soon as possible. You might need to receive follow-up care for several day's after you give birth. Your liver health will likely return to normal within a few weeks of giving birth.

Alcoholic Fatty Liver Disease (ALFD): Drinking a lot of alcohol damages the liver. When it's damaged, the liver can't break down fat properly. This can cause fat to build up, which is known as alcoholic fatty liver. Alcoholic fatty liver disease (ALFD) is the earliest stage of alcohol-related liver disease. If there's no inflammation or other complications along with the build-up of fat, the condition is known as simple alcoholic fatty liver.

Alcoholic Steatohepatitis (ASH): Alcoholic steatohepatitis (ASH) is a type of AFLD. It happens when a build-up of excess fat in the liver is accompanied by liver inflammation.This is also known as alcoholic hepatitis. If you have excess fat in your liver, your liver is inflamed, and you drink a lot of alcohol, your doctor may diagnose you with ASH.If it's not treated properly, ASH can cause scarring of your liver. Severe liver scarring is known as cirrhosis.It can lead to liver failure.To treat alcoholic fatty liver, it's important to avoid alcohol. If you have alcoholism, or alcohol use disorder, your doctor may recommend counseling or other treatments.

Risk Factors

Drinking high amounts of alcohol puts you at increased risk of developing fatty liver. You may also be at heightened risk if you:

- Are obese
- Have insulin resistance
- Have type 2 diabetes
- Have polycystic ovary syndrome
- Are pregnant
- Have a history of certain infections, such as hepatitis c
- Take certain medications, such as methotrexate (trexall), tamoxifen (nolvadex), amiodorone (pacerone), and valproic acid (depakote)
- Have high cholesterol levels
- Have high triglyceride levels
- Have high blood sugar levels
- Have metabolic syndrome

If you have a family history of fatty liver disease, you're more likely to develop it yourself.

Stages Of Fatty Liver

Fatty Liver Can Progress Through Four Stages:

- Simple fatty liver. There is a build-up of excess fat in the liver.
- Steatohepatitis. In addition to excess fat, there is inflammation in the liver.

- Fibrosis. Inflammation in the liver has caused scarring.
- Cirrhosis. Scarring of the liver has become widespread.

Cirrhosis is a potentially life-threatening condition that can cause liver failure.It may be irreversible. That's why it's so important to prevent it from developing in the first place.To help stop fatty liver from progressing and causing complications, follow your doctor's recommended treatment plan.

Prevention

To prevent fatty liver and its potential complications, it's important to follow a healthy lifestyle.

- Limit or avoid alcohol.
- Maintain a healthy weight.
- Eat a nutrient-rich diet that's low in saturated fats, trans fats, and refined carbohydrates.
- Take steps to control your blood sugar, triglyceride levels, and cholesterol levels.
- Follow your doctor's recommended treatment plan for diabetes, if you have it.
- Aim for at least 30 minutes of exercise most days of the week.

Liver Cancer

Liver cancer is cancer that occurs in the liver. The liver is the largest glandular organ in the body and performs various critical functions to keep the body free of toxins and harmful substances. It's located in the right upper quadrant of the abdomen, right below the ribs. The liver is responsible for producing bile, which is a substance that helps you digest fats, vitamins, and other nutrients. This vital organ also stores nutrients such as glucose, so that you remain nourished at times when you're not eating. It also breaks down medications and toxins.When cancer develops in the liver, it destroys liver cells and interferes with the ability of the liver to function normally. Liver cancer is generally classified as primary or secondary. Primary liver cancer begins in the cells of the liver.Secondary liver cancer develops when cancer cells from another organ spread to the liver. Unlike other cells in the body, cancer cells can break away from the primary site, or where the cancer began. The cells travel to other areas of the body through the bloodstream or the lymphatic system.Cancer cells eventually collect in another body organ and begin to grow there.

Different Types Of Primary Liver Cancer

The different types of primary liver cancer originate from the various cells that make up the liver. Primary liver cancer can start as a single lump growing in the liver, or it can start in many places within the liver at the same time. People with severe liver damage are more likely to have multiple cancer growth sites. The main types of primary liver cancer are:

Hepatocellular Carcinoma: Hepatocellular carcinoma (HCC), also known as hepatoma, is the most common type of liver cancer, accounting for 75 percent of all liver cancers. This condition develops in the hepatocytes, which are the predominant liver cells. It can spread from the liver to other parts of the body, such as the pancreas, intestines, and stomach. HCC is much more likely to occur in people who have severe liver damage due to alcohol abuse.

Cholangiocarcinoma: Cholangiocarcinoma, more commonly known as bile duct cancer, develops in the small, tube-like bile ducts in the liver. These ducts carry bile to the gallbladder to help with digestion. Bile duct cancer accounts for approximately 10 to 20 percent of all liver cancers. When the cancer begins in the section of the ducts inside the liver, it's called intrahepatic bile duct cancer.When the cancer begins in the section of the ducts outside the liver, it's called extrahepatic bile duct cancer.

Liver Angiosarcoma: Liver angiosarcoma is a rare form of liver cancer that begins in the blood vessels of the liver.This type of cancer tends to progress very quickly, so it's typically diagnosed at a more advanced stage.

Hepatoblastoma: Hepatoblastoma is an extremely rare type of liver cancer. It's nearly always found in children, especially those under age 3. With surgery and chemotherapy, the outlook for people with this type of cancer can be very good. When hepatoblastoma is detected in the early stages, the survival rate is higher than 90 percent.

Symptoms Of Liver Cancer

Many people don't experience symptoms in the early stages of primary liver cancer.When symptoms do appear, they may include:

- Abdominal discomfort, pain, and tenderness
- Yellowing of the skin and the whites of the eyes, which is called jaundice
- White, chalky stools
- Nausea

- Vomiting
- Bruising or bleeding easily
- Weakness
- Fatigue

People At Risk Of Liver Cancer

Doctors aren't sure why some people get liver cancer while others don't. However, there are certain factors that are known to increase the risk of developing liver cancer:

- Liver cancer is more common in people over age 50.
- A long-term hepatitis B or C infection can severely damage your liver. Hepatitis is spread from person-to-person through direct contact with the bodily fluids of an infected person, such as their blood or semen. It may also be passed from mother to child during childbirth. You can lower your risk for hepatitis B and C by using protection during sexual intercourse. There's also a vaccine that can protect you against hepatitis B.
- Having two or more alcoholic beverages every day over many years increases your risk for liver cancer.
- Cirrhosis is a form of liver damage in which healthy tissue is replaced by scarred tissue. A scarred liver can't function properly and may ultimately lead to numerous

complications, including liver cancer. Long-term alcohol abuse and hepatitis C are the most common causes of cirrhosis in the United States. The majority of Americans with liver cancer have cirrhosis before they develop liver cancer.

- Exposure to aflatoxin is a risk factor. Aflatoxin is a toxic substance produced by a type of mold that can grow on peanuts, grains, and corn. In the United States, food-handling laws limit widespread exposure to aflatoxin. Outside of the country, however, aflatoxin exposure can be high.
- Diabetes and obesity are also risk factors. People with diabetes tend to be overweight or obese, which can cause liver problems and increase risk for liver cancer.

Liver Cancer Diagnosis

The diagnosis of liver cancer begins with a medical history and a physical examination. Make sure to tell your doctor if you have a history of long-term alcohol abuse or a chronic hepatitis B or C infection. Diagnostic tests and procedures for liver cancer include the following:

- Liver function tests help your doctor determine the health of your liver by measuring levels of proteins, liver enzymes, and bilirubin in your blood.
- The presence of alpha-fetoprotein(AFP) in the blood can be a sign of liver cancer. This protein is usually only produced in the liver and yolk sac of babies before they're born. AFP production normally stops after birth.
- Abdominal CT or MRI scans produce detailed images of the liver and other organs in the abdomen. They can allow your doctor to pinpoint where a tumor is developing, determine its size, and assess whether it has spread to other organs.

Liver Biopsy: Another diagnostic test available is a liver biopsy. A liver biopsy involves removing a small piece of liver tissue. It's always done using anesthesia to prevent you from feeling any pain during the procedure. In most cases, a needle biopsy is performed. During this procedure, your doctor will insert a thin needle through your abdomen and into your liver to obtain a tissue sample. The sample is then examined under a microscope for signs of cancer. A liver biopsy might also be performed using a laparoscope, which is a thin, flexible tube with an attached camera. The camera allows your doctor to see what the liver looks like and to perform a more precise biopsy. The laparoscope is inserted through a small incision in the abdomen. If tissue samples from other organs are needed, your doctor will make a larger incision. This is called a laparotomy. If liver cancer is found, your doctor will determine the stage of the cancer.Staging describes the severity or extent of the cancer. It can help your doctor determine your treatment options and your outlook.

Liver Cancer Treatment

Treatment for liver cancer varies.It depends on:

- The Number, Size, And Location Of The Tumors In The Liver
- How Well The Liver Is Functioning
- Whether Cirrhosis Is Present
- Whether The Tumor Has Spread To Other Organs

Your specific treatment plan will be based on these factors. Liver cancer treatments may include the following:

Hepatectomy: A hepatectomy is performed to remove either a portion of the liver or all of the liver. This surgery is usually done when the cancer is confined to the liver.Over time, the remaining healthy tissue will regrow and replace the missing part.

Liver Transplant: A liver transplant involves replacing the entire diseased liver with a healthy liver from a suitable donor. A transplant can only be done if the cancer hasn't spread to other organs. Medicines to prevent rejection are given after the transplant.

Ablation: Ablation involves the use of heat or ethanol injections to destroy the cancer cells. It's performed using local anesthesia.This numbs the area to prevent you from feeling any pain.Ablation can help people who aren't candidates for surgery or a transplant.

Chemotherapy: Chemotherapy is an aggressive form of drug therapy that destroys cancer cells. The medications are injected intravenously or through a vein.In most cases, chemotherapy can be given as an outpatient treatment.Chemotherapy can be effective in treating liver cancer, but many people experience side effects during treatment, including vomiting, decreased appetite, and chills. Chemotherapy can also increase your risk of infection.

Radiation Therapy: Radiation therapy involves the use of high-energy radiation beams to kill cancer cells. It can be delivered by external beam radiation or by internal radiation. In external beam radiation, the radiation is aimed at the abdomen and chest. Internal radiation involves the use of a catheter to inject tiny radioactive spheres into the hepatic artery. The radiation then destroys the hepatic artery, a blood vessel that supplies blood to the liver.This decreases the amount of blood flowing to the tumor. When the hepatic artery is closed off, the portal vein continues to nourish the liver.

Targeted Therapy: Targeted therapy involves the use of medications that are designed to hit cancer cells where they're vulnerable. They decrease tumor growth and help shut down blood supply to the tumor. Sorafenib (Nexavar) has been approved as targeted therapy for people with liver cancer.Targeted therapy can be helpful for people who aren't candidates for a hepatectomy or liver transplant.However, targeted therapy can have significant side effects.

Embolization And Chemoembolization: Embolization and chemoembolization are surgical procedures. They're done to block off the hepatic artery. Your doctor will use small sponges or other particles to do this.This reduces the amount of blood flowing to the tumor.In chemoembolization, your doctor injects chemotherapy drugs into the hepatic artery before the particles are injected. The blockage created keeps the chemotherapy medications in the liver for a longer period.

Liver Cancer Prevention

Liver cancer can't always be prevented. However, you reduce your risk for liver cancer by taking steps to prevent the development of conditions that can lead to liver cancer.

Get the Hepatitis B Vaccine: There's a vaccine for hepatitis B that all children should receive. Adults who are at high risk for infection, such as those who abuse intravenous drugs, should also be vaccinated. The vaccination is usually given in a series of three injections over a period of six months.

Take Measures to Prevent Hepatitis C: There's no vaccine for hepatitis C, but you can reduce your risk of getting the infection by doing the following:

- Use protection. Always practice safe sex by using a condom with all of your sexual partners. You should never engage in unprotected sex unless you're certain your partner isn't infected with hepatitis or any other sexually transmitted infection.
- Don't use illegal drugs. Avoid using illegal drugs, particularly those that can be injected, such as heroin or cocaine. If you're unable to stop using drugs, make sure

to use a sterile needle each time you inject them. Never share needles with other people.
- Be cautious about tattoos and piercings. Go to a trustworthy shop whenever you get a piercing or tattoo. Ask employees about their safety practices and make sure they use sterile needles.

Reduce Your Risk Of Cirrhosis

You can lower your risk of cirrhosis by doing the following:

- If you drink alcohol, drink in moderation. Limiting the amount of alcohol you drink can help prevent liver damage. Women shouldn't drink more than one drink per day, and men shouldn't drink more than two drinks per day.
- Maintain a healthy weight. Exercising for 30 minutes at least three times per week can help you maintain your weight. Eating a balanced diet is also important for weight management. Make sure you incorporate lean protein, whole grains, and vegetables or fruit into most of your meals. If you need to lose weight, increase the amount of exercise you do each day and reduce the number of calories you consume. You may also want to consider meeting with a nutritionist. They can help you

create a meal plan and exercise routine that allow you to achieve your weight loss goals more quickly.

If you already have one of these conditions and you're concerned about your risk for liver cancer, talk to your doctor about a liver cancer screening.

Liver Detox Diet

Foods That Are Good For Your Liver

The liver is a powerhouse of an organ. It performs a variety of essential tasks, ranging from producing proteins, cholesterol and bile to storing vitamins, minerals and even carbohydrates. It also breaks down toxins like alcohol, medications and natural byproducts of metabolism. Keeping your liver in good shape is important for maintaining health.

Coffee

Coffee is one of the best beverages you can drink to promote liver health. Studies have shown that drinking coffee protects the liver from disease, even in those who already have problems with this organ. For example, studies have repeatedly shown that drinking coffee lowers the risk of cirrhosis, or permanent liver damage, in people with chronic liver disease. Drinking coffee may also reduce the risk of developing a common type of liver cancer, and it has positive effects on liver disease and inflammation. It's even associated with a lower risk of death in people with chronic liver disease, with the greatest benefits seen in those who drink at least three cups per day. These benefits seem to stem from its ability to prevent the buildup of fat and collagen, two of the main markers of liver disease. Coffee also decreases inflammation and increases levels of the antioxidant glutathione. Antioxidants neutralize harmful free radicals, which are produced naturally in the body and can cause damage to cells. While coffee has many health benefits, your liver, in particular, will thank you for that morning cup of joe.

Tea

Tea is widely considered to be beneficial for health, but evidence has shown that it may have particular benefits for the liver. One large Japanese study found that drinking 5–10 cups of green tea per day was associated with improved blood markers of liver health. A smaller study in non-alcoholic fatty liver disease (NAFLD) patients found drinking green tea high in antioxidants for 12 weeks improved liver enzyme levels and may also reduce oxidative stress and fat deposits in the liver. Furthermore, another review found that people who drank green tea were less likely to develop liver cancer. The lowest risk was seen in people who drank four or more cups per day. A number of mouse and rat studies have also demonstrated the beneficial effects of black and green tea extracts. For example, one study in mice found that black tea extract reversed many of the negative effects of a high-fat diet on the liver, as well as improved blood markers of liver health. Nevertheless, some people, especially those who have liver problems, should exercise caution before consuming green tea as a supplement. That's because there have been several reports of liver damage resulting from the use of supplements containing green tea extract.

Grapefruit

Grapefruit contains antioxidants that naturally protect the liver. The two main antioxidants found in grapefruit are naringenin and naringin. Several animal studies have found that both help protect the liver from injury. The protective effects of grapefruit are known to occur in two ways — by reducing inflammation and protecting cells. Studies have also shown that these antioxidants can reduce the development of hepatic fibrosis, a harmful condition in which excessive connective tissue builds up in the liver. This typically results from chronic inflammation. Moreover, in mice that were fed a high-fat diet, naringenin decreased the amount of fat in the liver and increased the number of enzymes necessary for burning fat, which can help prevent excess fat from accumulating. Lastly, in rats, naringin has been shown to improve the ability to metabolize alcohol and counteract some of alcohol's negative effects. Thus far, the effects of grapefruit or grapefruit juice itself, rather than its components, have not been studied. Additionally, almost all studies looking at the antioxidants in grapefruit have been conducted in animals. Nevertheless, the current evidence points to grapefruit being a good way to keep your liver healthy by fighting damage and inflammation.

Blueberries And Cranberries

Blueberries and cranberries both contain anthocyanins, antioxidants that give berries their distinctive colors. They've also been connected to many health benefits.Several animal studies have demonstrated that whole cranberries and blueberries, as well as their extracts or juices, can help keep the liver healthy. Consuming these fruits for 3–4 weeks protected the liver from damage. Additionally, blueberries helped increase immune cell response and antioxidant enzymes. Another experiment found that the types of antioxidants found commonly in berries slowed the development of lesions and fibrosis, the development of scar tissue, in the livers of rats. What's more, blueberry extract has even been shown to inhibit the growth of human liver cancer cells in test-tube studies. However, more studies are needed to determine if this effect can be replicated in the human body. Making these berries a regular part of your diet is a good way to make sure your liver is supplied with the antioxidants it needs to stay healthy.

Grapes

Grapes, especially red and purple grapes, contain a variety of beneficial plant compounds. The most famous one is resveratrol, which has a number of health benefits. Many animal studies have shown that grapes and grape juice can benefit the liver.Studies have found that they can have various benefits, including lowering inflammation, preventing damage and increasing antioxidant levels. A small study in humans with NAFLD showed that supplementing with grape seed extract for three months improved liver function. However, since grape seed extract is a concentrated form, you might not see the same effects from consuming whole grapes. More studies are needed before taking grape seed extract for the liver can be recommended. Nonetheless, the wide range of evidence from animal and some human studies suggests that grapes are a very liver-friendly food.

Prickly Pear

Prickly pear, known scientifically as Opuntia ficus-indica, is a popular type of edible cactus. Its fruit and juice are most commonly consumed. It has long been used in traditional medicine as a treatment for ulcers, wounds, fatigue and liver disease. A 2004 study in 55 people found that the extract of this plant reduced symptoms of a hangover. Participants experienced less nausea, dry mouth and lack of appetite and were half as likely to experience a severe hangover if they consumed the extract before drinking alcohol, which is detoxified by the liver. The study concluded these effects were due to a reduction in inflammation, which often occurs after drinking alcohol. Another study in mice found that consuming prickly pear extract helped normalize enzyme and cholesterol levels when consumed at the same time as a pesticide known to be harmful to the liver. Subsequent studies found similar results. A more recent study in rats sought to determine the effectiveness of prickly pear juice, rather than its extract, at combating the negative effects of alcohol. This study found that the juice decreased the amount of oxidative damage and injury to the liver after alcohol consumption and helped keep antioxidant and inflammation levels stable. More human studies are needed, especially using prickly pear fruit and juice, rather than extract. Nonetheless, the studies thus far have demonstrated that prickly pear has positive effects on the liver.

Beetroot Juice

Beetroot juice is a source of nitrates and antioxidants called betalains, which may benefit heart health and reduce oxidative damage and inflammation. It's reasonable to assume that eating beets themselves would have similar health effects. However, most studies use beetroot juice. You can juice beets yourself or buy beetroot juice from the store or online. Several rat studies have shown that beetroot juice reduces oxidative damage and inflammation in the liver, as well as increases natural detoxification enzymes. While animal studies look promising, similar studies have not been done in humans. Other beneficial health effects of beetroot juice have been observed in animal studies and replicated in human studies. However, more studies are needed to confirm the benefits of beetroot juice on liver health in humans.

Cruciferous Vegetables

Cruciferous vegetables like Brussels sprouts, broccoli and mustard greens are known for their high fiber content and distinctive taste. They are also high in beneficial plant compounds. Animal studies have shown Brussels sprouts and broccoli sprout extract increase levels of detoxification enzymes and protect the liver from damage. A study in human liver cells found that this effect remained even when Brussels sprouts were cooked. A recent study in men with fatty liver found that broccoli sprout extract, which is high in beneficial plant compounds, improved liver enzyme levels and decreased oxidative stress. The same study found that the broccoli sprout extract prevented liver failure in rats. Human studies are limited. But so far, cruciferous vegetables look promising as a beneficial food for liver health. Try lightly roasting them with garlic and lemon juice or balsamic vinegar to turn them into a tasty and healthy dish.

Nuts

Nuts are high in fats, nutrients — including the antioxidant vitamin E — and beneficial plant compounds. This composition is responsible for several health benefits, especially for heart health, but potentially also for the liver. One six-month observational study in 106 people with non-alcoholic fatty liver disease found eating nuts was associated with improved levels of liver enzymes. What's more, a second observational study found that men who ate small amounts of nuts and seeds had a higher risk of developing NAFLD than men who ate large amounts of nuts and seeds. While more high-quality studies are needed, preliminary data points to nuts being an important food group for liver health.

Fatty Fish

Fatty fish contain omega-3 fatty acids, which are healthy fats that reduce inflammation and have been associated with a lower risk of heart disease. The fats found in fatty fish are beneficial for the liver, as well. In fact, studies have shown that they help prevent fat from building up, keep enzyme levels normal, fight inflammation and improve insulin resistance. While consuming omega-3-rich fatty fish appears to be beneficial for your liver, adding more omega-3 fats to your diet is not the only thing to consider. The ratio of omega-3 fats to omega-6 fats is also important.Most Americans exceed the intake recommendations for omega-6 fats, which are found in many plant oils. An omega-6 to omega-3 ratio that is too high can promote the development of liver disease. Therefore, it's a good idea to reduce your intake of omega-6 fats, too.

Olive Oil

Olive oil is considered a healthy fat because of its many health benefits, including positive effects on heart and metabolic health. However, it also has positive effects on the liver. One small study in 11 people with NAFLD found that consuming one teaspoon (6.5 ml) of olive oil per day improved liver enzyme and fat levels. It also raised levels of a protein associated with positive metabolic effects. The participants also had less fat accumulation and better blood flow in the liver. Several more recent studies have found similar effects of olive oil consumption in humans, including less fat accumulation in the liver, improved insulin sensitivity and improved blood levels of liver enzymes.Fat accumulation in the liver is part of the first stage of liver disease. Therefore, olive oil's positive effects on liver fat, as well as other aspects of health, make it a valuable part of a healthy diet.

Foods To Help Fatty Liver Reversal

There are two major types of fatty liver disease alcohol-induced and nonalcoholic fatty liver disease. Fatty liver disease affects nearly one-third of American adults and is one of the leading contributors to liver failure.Nonalcoholic fatty liver disease is most commonly diagnosed in those who are obese or sedentary and those who eat a highly processed diet.One of the main ways to treat fatty liver disease, regardless of type, is with diet. As the name suggests, fatty liver disease means you have too much fat in your liver. In a healthy body, the liver helps to remove toxins and produces bile, the digestive protein. Fatty liver disease damages the liver and prevents it from working as well as it should.In general, the diet for fatty liver disease includes:

- Lots of fruits and vegetables
- High-fiber plants like legumes and whole grains
- Very little added sugar, salt, trans fat, refined carbohydrates, and saturated fat
- No alcohol

A low-fat, reduced-calorie diet can help you lose weight and reduce the risk of fatty liver disease. Ideally, if you're overweight, you would aim to lose at least 10 percent of your body weight.

Foods And Drinks That You Should Eat For A Fatty Liver

Here are a few foods to include in your healthy liver diet:

- Coffee to lower abnormal liver enzymes: Studies have shown that coffee drinkers with fatty liver disease have less liver damage than those who don't drink this caffeinated beverage. Caffeine appears to lower the amount of abnormal liver enzymes of people at risk for liver diseases.
- Greens to prevent fat buildup: Broccoli is shown to help prevent the buildup of fat in the liver in mice. Eating more greens, like spinach, Brussels sprouts, and kale, can also help with general weight loss.
- Tofu to reduce fat buildup: A University of Illinois study on rats found that soy protein, which is contained in foods like tofu, may reduce fat buildup in the liver. Plus, tofu is low in fat and high in protein.
- Fish for inflammation and fat levels: Fatty fish such as salmon, sardines, tuna, and trout are high in omega-3

fatty acids. Omega-3 fatty acids can help improve liver fat levels and bring down inflammation.
- Oatmeal for energy: Carbohydrates from whole grains like oatmeal give your body energy. Their fiber content also fills you up, which can help you maintain your weight.
- Walnuts to improve the liver: These nuts are high in omega-3 fatty acids. Research finds that people with fatty liver disease who eat walnuts have improved liver function tests.
- Avocado to help protect the liver: Avocados are high in healthy fats, and research suggests they contain chemicals that might slow liver damage. They're also rich in fiber, which can help with weight control.
- Milk and other low-fat dairy to protect from damage: Dairy is high in whey protein, which may protect the liver from further damage, according to a 2011 study in rats.
- Sunflower seeds for antioxidants: These nutty-tasting seeds are high in vitamin E, an antioxidant that may protect the liver from further damage.
- Olive oil for weight control: This healthy oil is high in omega-3 fatty acids. It's healthier for cooking than

margarine, butter, or shortening. Research finds that olive oil helps to lower liver enzyme levels and control weight. Try this liver-friendly take on a traditional Mexican dish.

- Garlic to help reduce body weight: This herb not only adds flavor to food, but experimental studies also show that garlic powder supplements may help reduce body weight and fat in people with fatty liver disease.

- Green tea for less fat absorption: Data supports that green tea can help interfere with fat absorption, but the results aren't conclusive yet. Researchers are studying whether green tea can reduce fat storage in the liver and improve liver function. But green tea also has many benefits, from lowering cholesterol to aiding with sleep.

Foods To Avoid If You Have A Fatty Liver

There are definitely foods you should avoid or limit if you have fatty liver disease. These foods generally contribute to weight gain and increasing blood sugar.

- Alcohol. Alcohol is a major cause of fatty liver disease as well as other liver diseases.

- Added sugar. Stay away from sugary foods such as candy, cookies, sodas, and fruit juices. High blood sugar increases the amount of fat buildup in the liver.
- Fried foods. These are high in fat and calories.
- Salt. Eating too much salt can make your body hold on to excess water. Limit sodium to less than 1,500 milligrams per day.
- White bread, rice, and pasta. White usually means the flour is highly processed, which can raise your blood sugar more than whole grains due to a lack of fiber.
- Red meat. Beef and deli meats are high in saturated fat.

Meal Menu

Breakfast

- 8 oz. hot oatmeal mixed with 2 tsp. almond butter and 1 sliced banana
- 1 cup coffee with low-fat or skim milk

Lunch

- spinach salad with balsamic vinegar and olive oil dressing
- 3 oz. grilled chicken
- 1 small baked potato

- 1 cup cooked broccoli, carrots, or other vegetable
- 1 apple
- 1 glass of milk

Snack

- 1 tbsp. peanut butter on sliced apples or 2 tbsp. hummus with raw veggies

Dinner

- Small mixed-bean salad
- 3 oz. Grilled salmon
- 1 cup cooked broccoli
- 1 whole-grain roll
- 1 cup mixed berries
- 1 glass of milk

Recipes

5-Ingredient Liver Detox Juice

Ingredients

- 1 beet, scrubbed

- one handful of greens, washed (dandelion greens are very good for the liver if you are ok with the bitter taste)
- 1 apple
- 1 cucumber, peeled
- 1 lemon, peeled
- Optional 1 scoop Superfood Turmeric

Instructions

- Juice all ingredients, stir and enjoy!

Dr. Group's Liver Cleanse Soup

Ingredients

- 3 cups filtered/purified water
- 1 cup organic vegetable broth
- 2 organic beets (peeled + diced)
- 2 organic carrots (sliced)
- 2 cups organic broccoli (chopped)
- 10 cloves organic garlic (freshly crushed)
- 1 organic onion (diced)
- 1/2 organic lemon (freshly squeezed)
- 2 organic bay leaves
- 1/2 teaspoon Himalayan pink salt

- 1/2 teaspoon organic ground turmeric
- 1/2 teaspoon organic dried oregano
- 1/2 teaspoon organic ground black pepper

Instructions

Prepare the veggies:

- Slice/Dice/Cut the beets, carrots, broccoli, and onions to the size of your preference.

Prepare the soup:

- Add all the ingredients for the soup to a medium-size pot and bring to a boil.
- Lower the heat and simmer on low heat for approximately 1 hour, or until the veggies are soft.
- Add extra water or veggie broth if needed and adjust seasonings to your preference.

Beet Kvass

Ingredients

- 3-4 small raw beets or 1 large raw beet, cut into 2-inch pieces
- 1 tablespoon Celtic sea salt

Instructions

- Place the beets in a 2-quart glass or ceramic pitcher. Cover with water and stir in the sea salt. Cover with a clean cloth and place in a dark cool place for 3 days. After 3 days, remove the beets and store the kvass in the fridge. It will keep for about 2 weeks.

Liver Cleansing Juice

Ingredients

- 2 stalks celery
- 1/2 bunch spinach
- 2 medium carrots
- 1 small beet
- 1-inch ginger root
- 1 small lemon
- 1 medium apple
- 2 ml Livatrex drops Liver cleansing herbs
- 2 medium cucumbers optional
- stevia to taste optional
- cinnamon optional

Instructions

- Peel the ginger, beetroot and lemon.
- Run the celery, spinach, carrots, beetroot, cucumbers, lemon, ginger, and apple through a juicer.
- Mix and taste. You can add a few drops of stevia to add sweetness (optional), or add another apple to the recipe.
- If you like cinnamon flavor, you may add a dash of cinnamon. This works very well in this juice recipe.
- Add 2 ml Livatrex
- Drink immediately.

Mean Green Detox Juice

Detoxification is a daily process. It is essential that we support our liver and all elimination organs with high-quality foods and specific nutrients. This will increase our body's ability to eliminate the toxins and chemicals it comes in contact with, and will help to support our health and overall longevity.

Tools

- Juicer or blender

Ingredients

- 4 large dandelion leaves

- 4 cups arugula
- 3 celery stalks
- 2 large broccoli stalks
- 2 carrots
- 1 lemon (with peel on)
- ½ a grapefruit

Instructions

- Process all ingredients through a juicer. Alternatively, if you have a high-speed blender, you can make this into a smoothie.
- Be sure to add enough water to blend your ingredients, and feel free to pour the mix through a sieve to strain out the fiber.

Conclusion

Lifestyle changes are the first-line treatment for fatty liver disease.Depending on your current condition and lifestyle habits.

Printed in Great Britain
by Amazon